WHAT IT MEANS TO BE A
Nurse

A CELEBRATION OF THE HUMOR, HEART, AND HEROES OF EVERY HOSPITAL

The Creator of
SNARKYNURSES

ADAMS MEDIA

NEW YORK   LONDON   TORONTO   SYDNEY   NEW DELHI

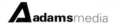

Adams Media
An Imprint of Simon & Schuster, Inc.
100 Technology Center Drive
Stoughton, MA 02072

First Adams Media hardcover edition April 2021

ADAMS MEDIA and colophon are trademarks of Simon & Schuster.

For information about special discounts for bulk purchases, please contact Simon & Schuster Special Sales at 1-866-506-1949 or business@simonandschuster.com.

The Simon & Schuster Speakers Bureau can bring authors to your live event. For more information or to book an event contact the Simon & Schuster Speakers Bureau at 1-866-248-3049 or visit our website at www.simonspeakers.com.

Interior design by Colleen Cunningham, Erin Alexander, Stephanie Hannus, Alaya Howard, Julia Jacintho, Sylvia McArdle, Victor Watch
Interior images © Getty Images; 123RF

Manufactured in the U.S.A.

10 9 8 7 6 5 4 3 2

Library of Congress Cataloging-in-Publication Data
Title: What it means to be a nurse / The creator of snarkynurses.
Description: First Adams Media hardcover edition. | Avon, Massachusetts: Adams Media, 2021. | Series: What it means.
Identifiers: LCCN 2020034988 | ISBN 9781507215340 (hc) | ISBN 9781507215357 (ebook)
Subjects: LCSH: Nursing--Humor. | Nurses--Anecdotes.
Classification: LCC RT61 . W44 2021 | DDC 610.73--dc23
LC record available at https://lccn.loc.gov/2020034988

ISBN 978-1-5072-1534-0
ISBN 978-1-5072-1535-7 (ebook)

Dedication

To my mom—
thank you for everything, especially for
instilling that twisted sense of humor!

And to my sugar bean—
perhaps someday you will see this and think
your mom was once kind of awesome.

Introduction

Do you hear call lights, IV pumps, and telemetry alarms in your sleep?

Did your patient just get out of bed without assistance for the seventy-seventh time this shift?

Despite the wild, eye-rolling moments, would you still choose nursing time and time again?

If so, you're clearly a nurse!

Nursing is likely one of the biggest loves of your life. You see life, death, and everything in between. While you may have started out choosing nursing as a career, eventually it becomes part of who you ARE. You live for moments when a parent finally holds their baby in their arms, a treatment plan works, or your patient laughs for the first time in literally days…even if it was because you tripped over your own clogs while walking into their room.

These moments and so many more are what make this profession so fulfilling. Nursing isn't all hilariously awesome coworkers and patients who know better than to use their call light excessively, so in those more challenging times, it's important to remember nurses are in this together. That's where *What It Means to Be a Nurse* comes in!

Within these pages you'll find more than 150 entries which are designed to pour some sunshine into your day when you need it the most, but also to make you laugh and say "Remember that one time…" to your nurse friends. Both humorous and inspiring, they serve as a reminder of why you chose nursing and why the nursing world needs YOU!

Now grab your nursing mug (you know you have one), fill it with your favorite caffeinated beverage (or wine), and dive into this celebration of nursing!

There may be days I contemplate a different career, but ultimately,

I KNOW NURSING IS FOR ME AND I AM FOR NURSING.

♥ ◄

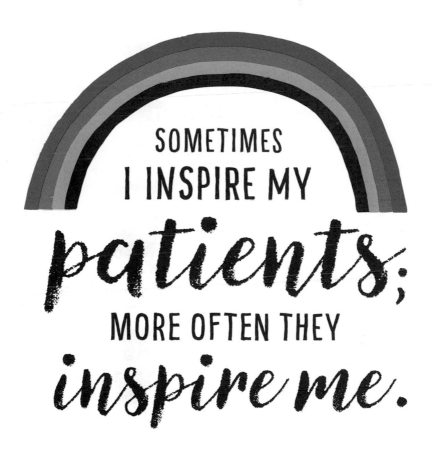

SOMETIMES
I INSPIRE MY
patients;
MORE OFTEN THEY
inspire me.

Hello
my name is

"NURRRRSSE!"

Together

WE ALL WORK HARD

for the

BEST
POSSIBLE
OUTCOMES.

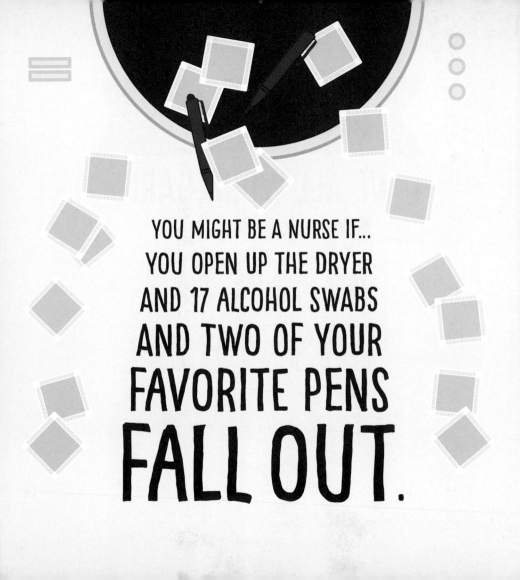

THE THINGS
YOU ARE
passionate
ABOUT ARE
NOT RANDOM,
they are
your calling.

—FABIENNE FREDRICKSON, FOUNDER OF BOLDHEART

Three words every nurse
loves hearing during
a coworker's report:

"I'm back
tomorrow."

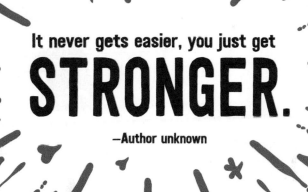

It never gets easier, you just get

STRONGER.

—Author unknown

ADVOCACY

the #1 priority for all nurses.

WHEN YOU'RE A NURSE, YOU KNOW *that* EVERY DAY YOU WILL TOUCH A LIFE *or a* LIFE WILL TOUCH YOURS.

—AUTHOR UNKNOWN

When your manager rolls by and asks how you're doing:

"I'M FINE, IT'S FINE, EVERYTHING'S FINE!"

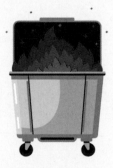

NARRATOR:

"EVERYTHING WAS NOT FINE."

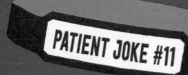

STRENGTH

HUMOR

TEAMWORK

COMPASSION

ADVOCATE

A work OF art
TO A nurse
IS getting that
18 GAUGE IV ON THE
FIRST TRY
AND dressing it
beautifully.

On those really
tough days,
don't forget...

miracles
happen.

WHAT INSPIRES A NURSE TO MOVE AT THE SPEED OF LIGHT?

A BED ALARM...

OR FRESH COFFEE IN THE BREAKROOM.

I've learned that people will *forget what you said*, people will *forget what you did*, but

people will never forget *how you made them feel.*

—Maya Angelou, poet

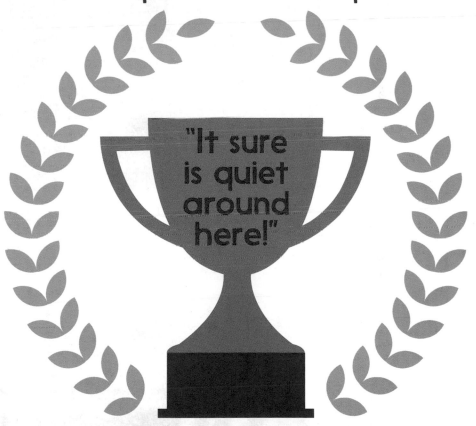

MURPHY'S LAW OF NURSING

#25

AS SOON AS YOU HAVE
GOWNED, GLOVED, MASKED,
AND WALKED INTO YOUR
PATIENT'S ROOM, YOU'LL
REMEMBER THREE OTHER
THINGS YOU NEEDED TO GET.

THE *best way* TO
find yourself
IS TO
lose yourself
IN THE service
of others.

—MAHATMA GANDHI,
lawyer, politician, and social activist

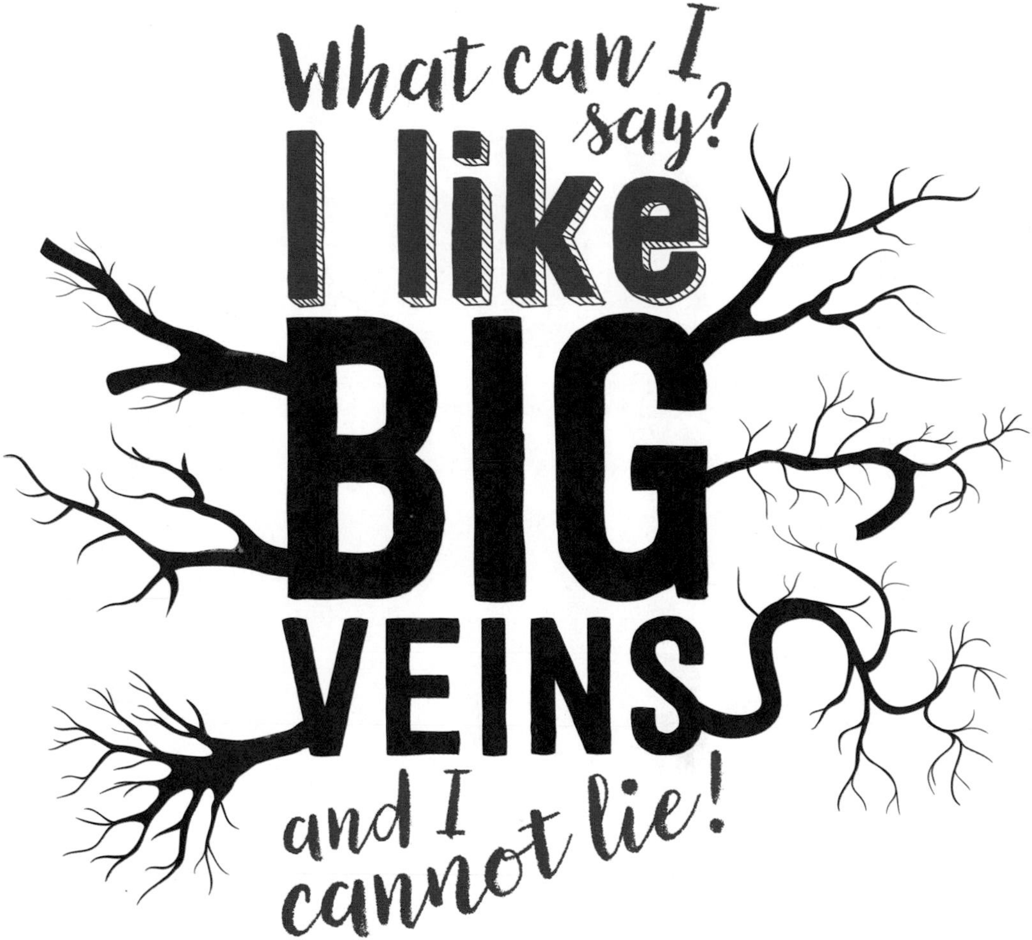
What can I say?
I like BIG VEINS
and I cannot lie!

Sometimes *the* BIGGEST GIFT *from a patient* *is a* SIMPLE "THANK YOU"

I don't know about you... but I find this HUMERUS.

It doesn't *matter* WHO you are, I will *take care* of YOU with a *devoted* ♥

My best friend's name is Pam.
She's pretty low-key and great to be around.

Lorazepam.

Diazepam.

Clonazepam.

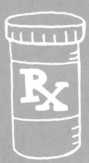

"A hero is an ordinary individual who finds the **STRENGTH to PERSEVERE and ENDURE** in spite of overwhelming obstacles."

—Christopher Reeve, actor

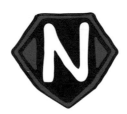

SOME OF THE
best friends
YOU WILL HAVE
ARE YOUR
coworkers.

THERE ARE NO
FRIENDSHIPS LIKE
*nurse
friendships.*

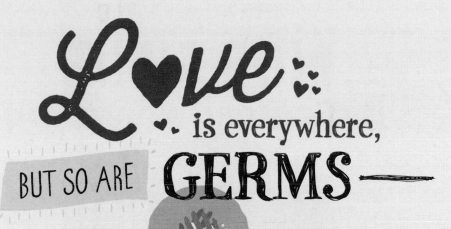

Love is everywhere, BUT SO ARE GERMS—

WASH YOUR HANDS PLEASE!

NURSING

is a career where you

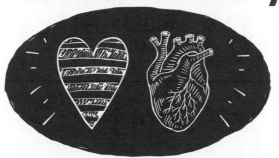

understand both
HEARTS.

NURSES...
SINGLE-HANDEDLY
KEEPING THE
ECONOMY AFLOAT
BY BUYING
CUTE SCRUBS
AND BADGE REELS.

I'M NOT TELLING YOU
IT'S GOING TO BE *easy.*
I'M TELLING YOU
IT'S GOING TO BE
worth it.

—Art Williams, insurance executive

You say
coffee,
I say
stat!

YOU MIGHT BE A NURSE IF...
YOU SURVIVED A 12-HOUR SHIFT ON graham crackers AND ginger ale FROM THE NUTRITION ROOM

MURPHY'S LAW OF NURSING

#32

WHENEVER YOU FINALLY
HAVE TIME TO PEE,
EVERY BATHROOM WILL
BE OCCUPIED.

Nursing hide-and-seek:

searching for a

LITTLE WHITE PILL

among the bedsheets.

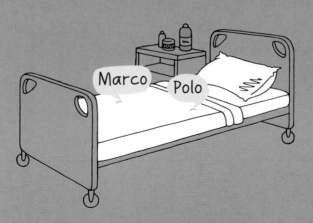

Just when you think
you've got it all together...

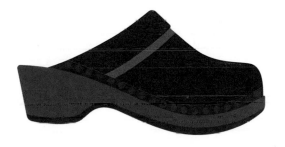

you trip and almost break
a cankle in your clogs.

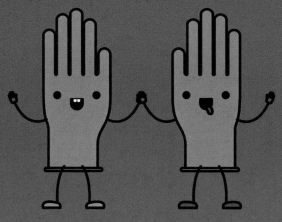

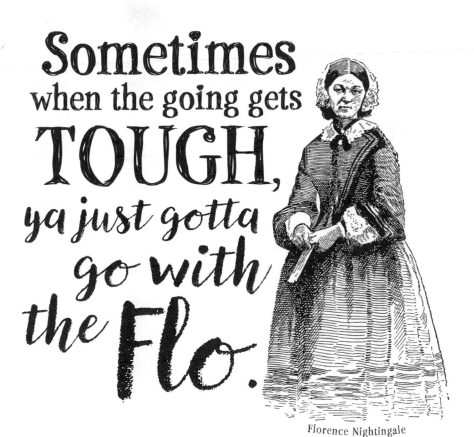

Sometimes when the going gets TOUGH, ya just gotta go with the Flo.

Florence Nightingale

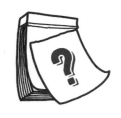

EIGHT TIMES OUT OF TEN I ASK MY PATIENT WHAT DAY IT IS AND DON'T EVEN KNOW THE ANSWER MYSELF.

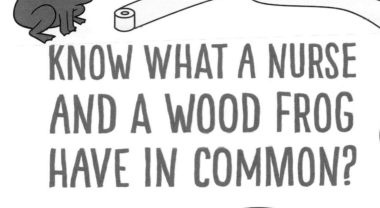

KNOW WHAT A NURSE AND A WOOD FROG HAVE IN COMMON?

THEY CAN BOTH HOLD **THEIR BLADDER** A REALLY LONG TIME.

It only takes one kind, thankful, and fun-loving patient to erase so many hard days.

Nothing beats the satisfaction of taking off your **compression socks** after twelve hours of pounding the hospital pavement.

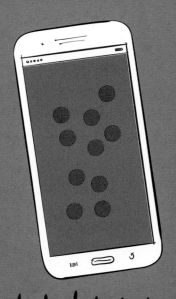

YOU MIGHT BE A NURSE IF...

YOU'VE RECEIVED TEXTS FROM FRIENDS AND FAMILY
ASKING YOU TO EXAMINE A RASH.

Are you even a nurse if you haven't heard **CALL LIGHTS** going off in your sleep?

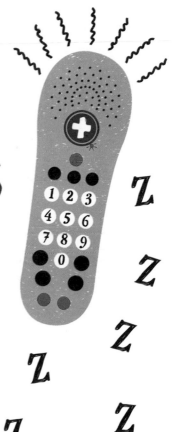

Always trust your instinct and advocate accordingly.

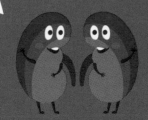

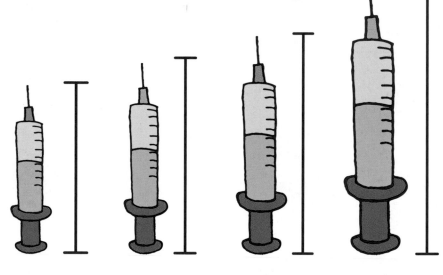

TO ERR IS HUMAN.

Every nurse has made a mistake; it's about how you *move forward* and *improve your practice* from there.

NURSES
ASSESS, advocate, educate, encourage, inspire, empathize, LEAD, respect, and innovate.

Know what day it is?

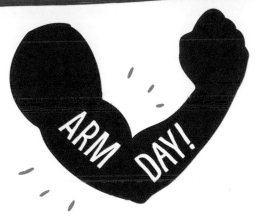

ARM DAY!

TWO SETS of reconstituting
piperacillin-tazobactam,
THREE SETS overhead IV fluid lifts,
and **INFINITE SETS** of turning,
lifting, and boosting patients.

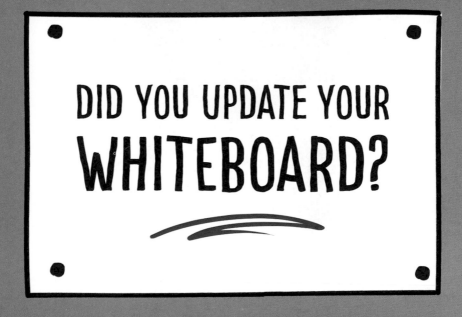

SOMETHING YOU CAN ALWAYS COUNT ON...

the pharmacy

WILL BE REFILLING MEDICATIONS
WHEN YOU NEED A MED

STAT.

KNOW WHAT NEVER FAILS?

The moment you walk out of an isolation room

and remove your **PPE**, the IV pump will

start singing the song of its people.

Even if you don't think you made a difference,

YOU DID.

PURE JOY

is finishing your shift (AND) still having all your favorite pens.

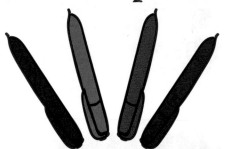

Nothing is more

REWARDING

than stepping up
to advocate for
your patient when they
are unable to do it
themselves.

I'm sorry, I can't because:

A
I'm on call.

B
I work tomorrow.

C
I'd rather sleep.

D
I have to go to my brother's best friend's hamster's funeral.

Telemetry:

where you can tell if your patient is up to no good
SIMPLY BY THEIR EKG TRACING.

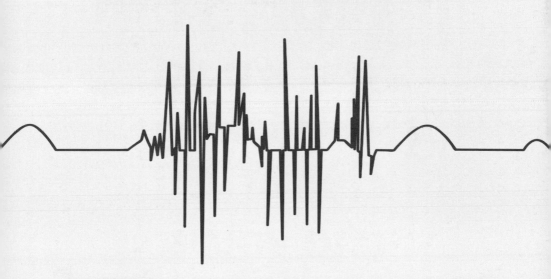

Strive to be
the kind of
NURSE
you would
want taking
care of you
and yours.

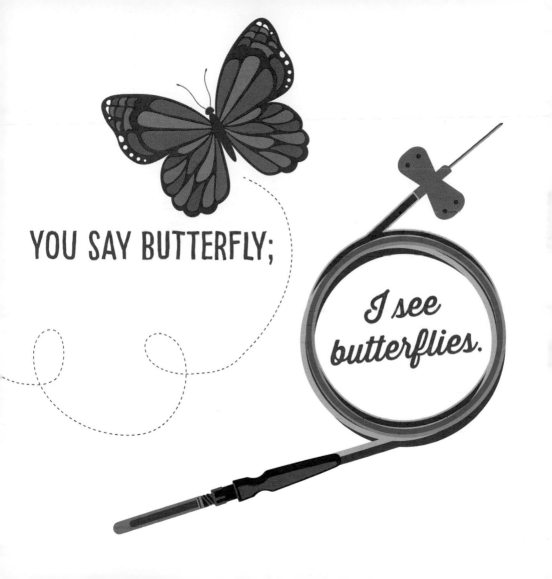

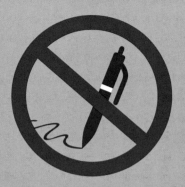

Nurses may share
tips and tricks to
make your shift easier
but don't ask to
borrow their pen.

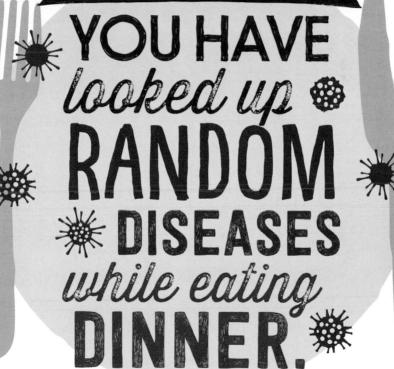

The magic of nursing lies in the little things:

Seeing your patient succeed.

Mastering a skill that you've struggled with.

Making lifelong friends.

Laughing about the absurdity of this profession.

A NURSE'S MEMORY IN A NUTSHELL:

You'll remember your patient's
entire medical history but get to
the supply room and forget four
of the five things you needed.

True
NURSING MAGIC

IS

WHEN YOU CAN MAKE A
patient laugh
DESPITE THEIR CURRENT SITUATION.

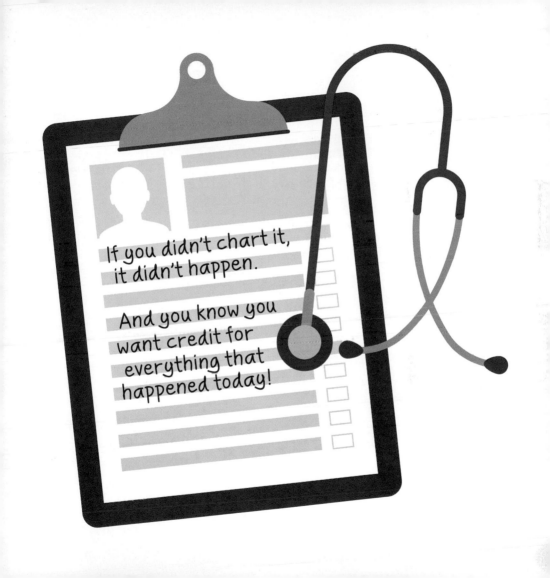

» NEVER »
UNDERESTIMATE
YOUR ABILITY TO
help a patient feel safe
AND
well taken care of.

Sometimes it's the little things that count, like full moons and Friday the 13th falling on your days off.

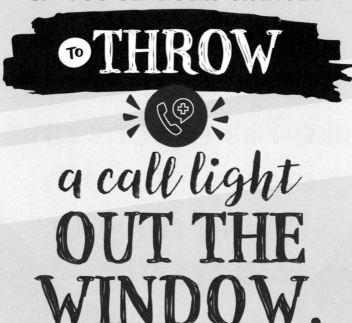

RAISE YOUR HAND
IF YOU'VE EVER WANTED
TO **THROW**
a call light
OUT THE
WINDOW.

MAY YOU ALWAYS HAVE THE

enthusiasm OF

A NEW GRAD NURSE

AND THE

HUMOR,

wisdom, and

UNFLAPPABLE

PRESENCE OF

A 30-YEAR NURSE.

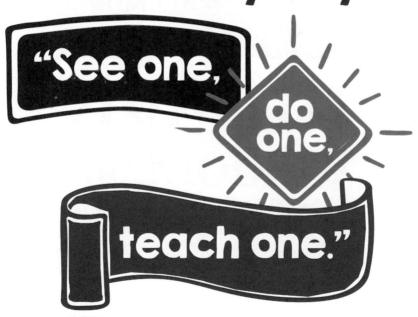

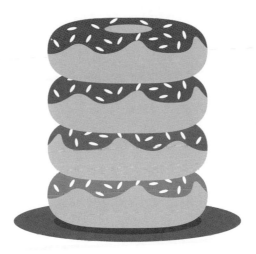

SOMETIMES YOU JUST NEED A PILE OF

doughnuts

TO SHOW UP ON THE BREAKROOM TABLE.

have you tried turning it off and on again?

Love,
adenosine

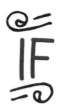

IF
nurses could
write orders:

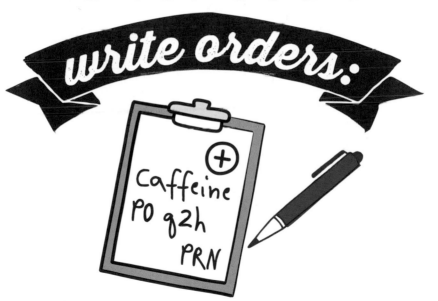

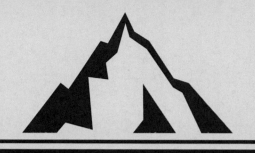

REMEMBER:
NURSES
ARE LIKE
ICEBERGS.

AT ANY ONE TIME,
YOU ARE ONLY
SEEING ABOUT
1/5 OF WHAT THEY
ARE ACTUALLY DOING.

—IAN MILLER, ER NURSE

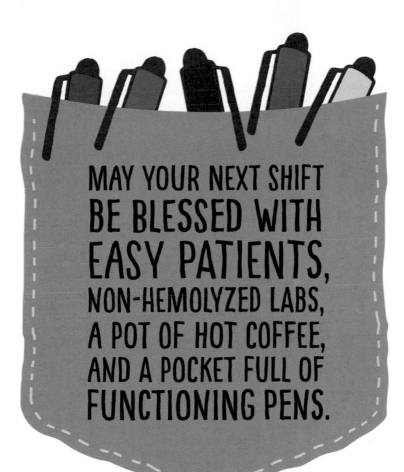

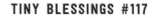

TINY BLESSINGS #117

*When you see
a ventricular tachycardia
alarm and run in to find
your patient brushing
their teeth!*

When I think about all the patients and their loved ones I have worked with over the years, I know most of them don't remember me, nor I them. But I do know that I gave a little piece of myself to each of them, and they to me, and those threads make up the tapestry that is my career in nursing.

—Donna Wilk Cardillo, RN and author

No one understands the frustration of an IV pump

SCREAMING

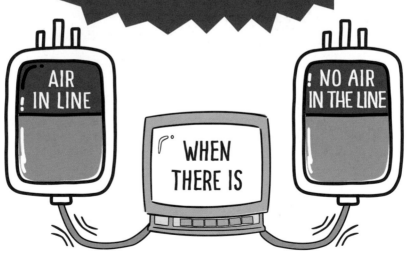

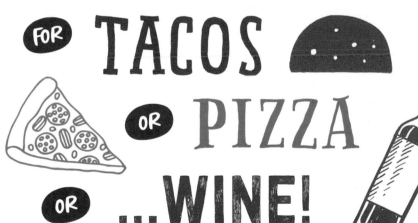

Friendly reminder:

Unless there's an emergency,

NO RUNNING & NO YELLING

RAISE YOUR HAND IF YOU'VE EVER FELT

PERSONALLY VICTIMIZED

BY A CHRISTMAS TREE.

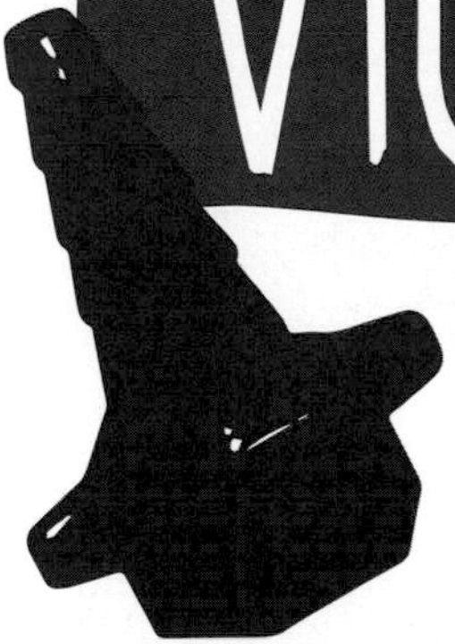

Sometimes the MOST "DIFFICULT" PATIENTS are the M♥ST REWARDING -TO- work with.

You might be a nurse if...

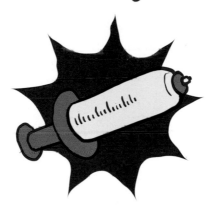

YOU KNOW THE
MAGICAL POWERS OF A
NORMAL SALINE FLUSH.

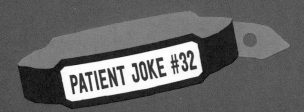

SHIFT CHANGE
might be my
ABSOLUTE
FAVORITE
time of day.

Once a nurse, always a nurse.

No matter where you go or what you do, you can never truly get out of nursing.

It's like the Mafia...YOU KNOW TOO MUCH.

—DEB GAULDIN, RN

HOW TO MAKE
A PATIENT HAPPY 101

1. Warm blankets
2. Turkey sandwiches
3. Ginger ale
4. Functioning TV
5. Repeat steps 1-4, especially 1

Always remember
your first
NURSE MENTOR
and aspire to be
like her or him.

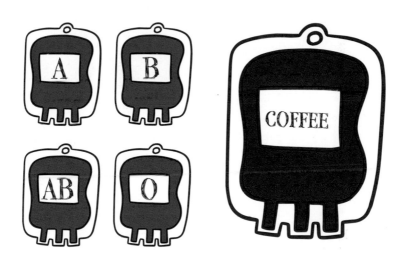

Which would you choose?

A

A breakroom full of delicious snacks and coffee and the ability to actually take a break!

B

All A&Ox4 independent patients.

A computer and mouse that are fast and fully functional.

Never having to wait for meds from the pharmacy.

☑ WAKE UP,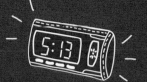

☑ THROW ON THOSE SCRUBS,

☑ FIND YOUR CAFFEINE,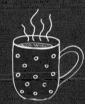

AND

☑ BE AWESOME!

MURPHY'S LAW OF NURSING

THE POOP WILL
ALMOST ALWAYS MISS
THE CHUX PAD DESPITE
YOUR BEST EFFORTS.

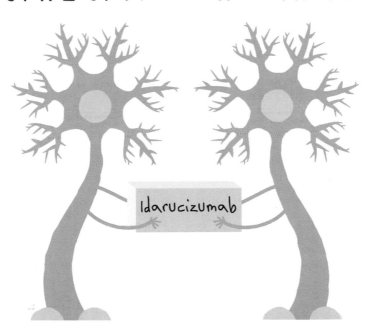

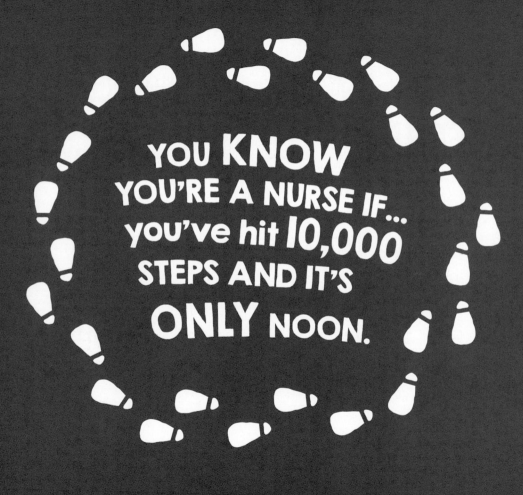
YOU KNOW YOU'RE A NURSE IF... you've hit 10,000 STEPS AND IT'S ONLY NOON.

MURPHY'S LAW OF NURSING

#59

YOU'LL FINISH YOUR
CHARTING AND REALIZE
YOU'RE IN THE WRONG
PATIENT'S CHART.

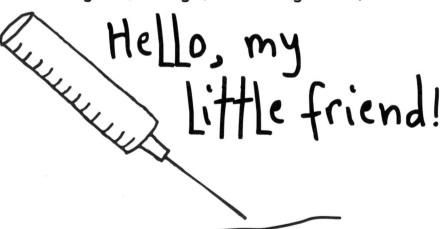

When you finally find a tiny vein for an IV:

Hello, my Little friend!

Nursing is a career where people from many **DIFFERENT BACKGROUNDS** come together *FOR* the same common goal: *to help people.*

TOP SIX NURSING WANTS:

MORE VACATION.

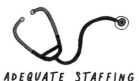

ADEQUATE STAFFING.

DELICIOUS POTLUCKS.

COFFEE. AT. ALL. TIMES.

KIND PATIENTS.

TO HAVE YOUR BESTIES WORKING
WITH YOU EVERY SHIFT.

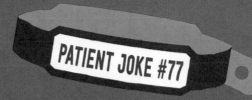

COWORKERS who have a **GREAT WORK ETHIC** and a **SENSE OF HUMOR** are the best!

MURPHY'S LAW OF NURSING

YOU'LL GET YOUR
PATIENT SETTLED BACK
INTO BED AND THEY'LL
WANT TO GET OUT AGAIN.

There's no **innovation** like **nurse innovation** at 2 a.m. when supply doesn't have what you need and you gotta *make it work!*

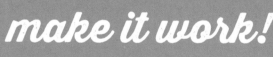

There are **4** types of people during a **CODE BLUE—** which are you?

1 YASSS! GET ME IN THERE!

2 I'll take care of the other patients!

3 Wait, there was a code blue?

4 ANYONE NEED A GLUCOMETER?

Nursing pet peeve #7:

Tattoos, shirts, stickers...
OKAY, BASICALLY
anything
WITH AN EKG RHYTHM
that doesn't actually look
like a real rhythm.

America's nurses

are the

beating heart

of our

MEDICAL SYSTEM.

—BARACK OBAMA,
44TH PRESIDENT OF THE UNITED STATES

NURSES ARE THERE WHEN the last breath is taken, AND NURSES ARE THERE WHEN the first breath is taken. ALTHOUGH IT IS MORE ENJOYABLE to celebrate the birth, IT IS JUST AS IMPORTANT to comfort in death.

—Christine Bell, author

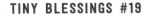

TINY BLESSINGS #19

When your patient's electrolyte labs come back within normal range and you don't have to replace them!

WHAT I SAID:

WHAT IT ACTUALLY MEANS:

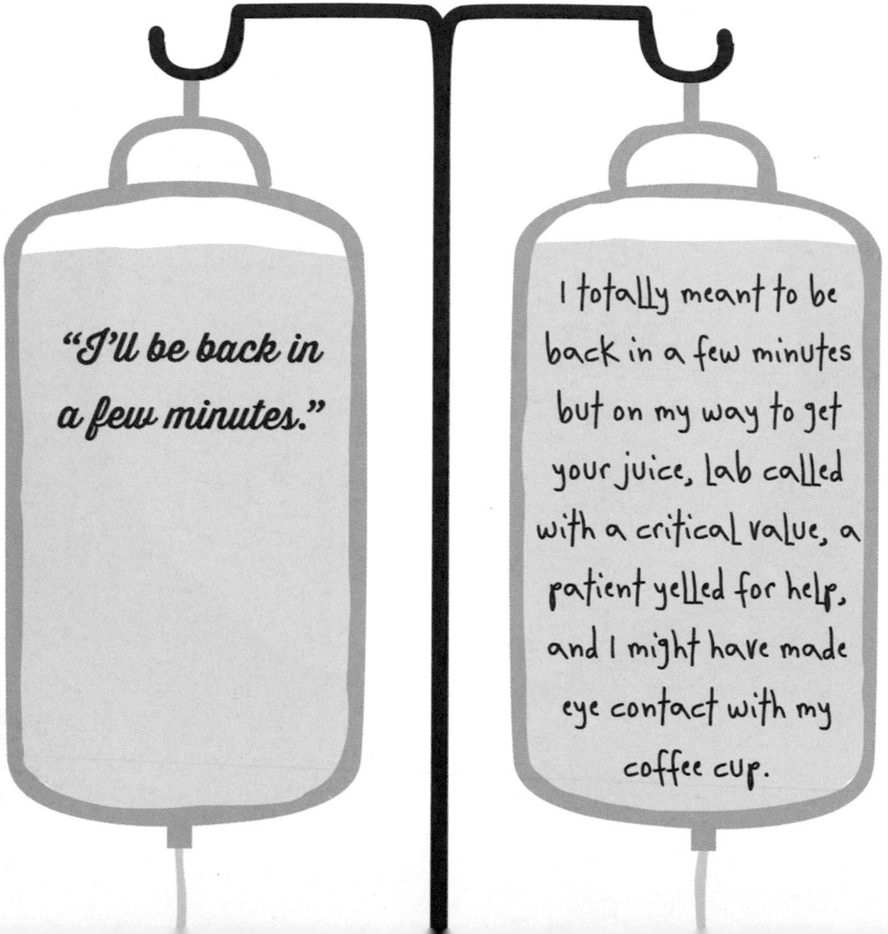

DOCTOR'S ORDERS THAT MAKE YOU GROAN

#7

Give
120mg
furosemide

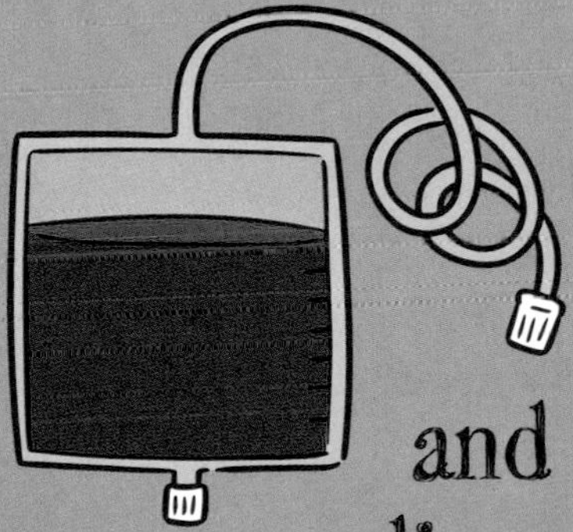

and
discontinue
catheter.

Nurses should support 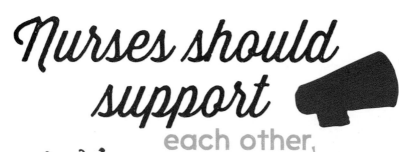 each other,

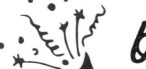 *be kind* to one another,

lift each other up when times are tough,

& empower one another.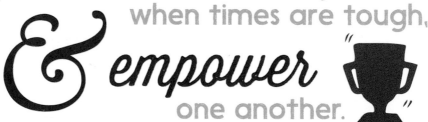

WORK ALL DAY: EAT NOTHING.

GET OFF WORK: INHALE BOAT-
LOAD OF CARBS BEFORE FALLING
ASLEEP 15 MINUTES LATER.

The bladder scanner,
pill crusher,
and EKG machine:

ALL HARDER TO FIND THAN WALDO.

Nurses

—one of the few *blessings* of being ill.

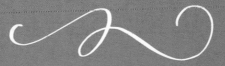

—Sara Moss-Wolfe, occupation unknown

TWO POSITIVES TO CRYING IN THE BATHROOM DURING AN OVERWHELMING DAY:

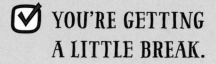 YOU'RE GETTING A LITTLE BREAK.

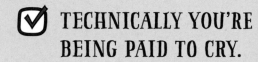 TECHNICALLY YOU'RE BEING PAID TO CRY.

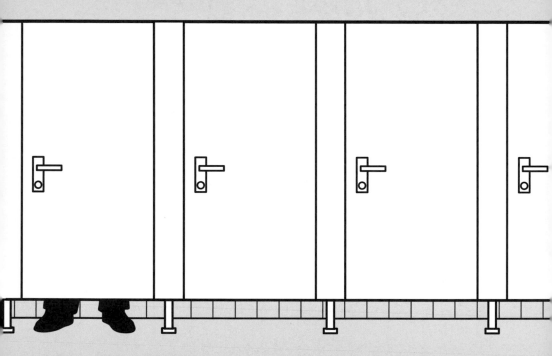

There's no satisfaction

like when the INTERN says

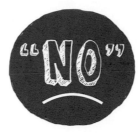

but the ATTENDING says

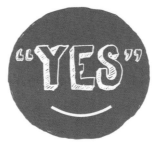

You know you're a nurse if...

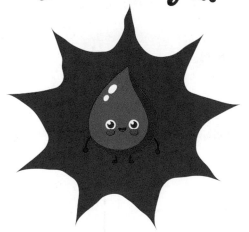

YOU FEEL A LIQUID LAND ON YOUR SHOE AND SOAK INTO YOUR SOCK AND YOU HOPE IT'S JUST URINE.

I'M SORRY TO SAY,
BUT WE ARE PROBABLY
GOING TO HAVE TO
DRAW SOME BLOOD.

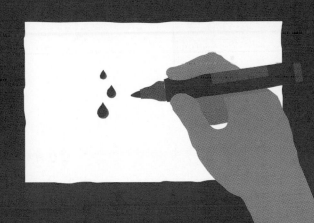

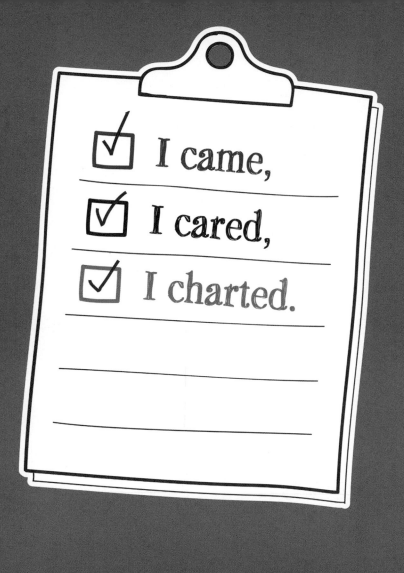

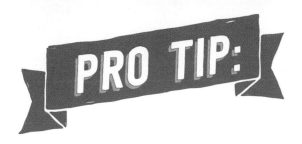

PRO TIP:

You can't get an admission if no one can find you!

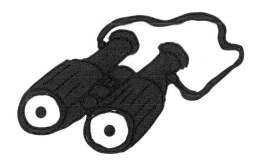

JUUUUUST KIDDING!

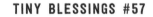

TINY BLESSINGS #57

When your patient's blood sugar is just below the level to give sliding scale insulin!

STRANGE THINGS NURSES FIND THEMSELVES SAYING:

"Whoa! That wound is so cool!"

"Have I peed today?"

"Where's the lube?"

"I wonder if I can pull off those cute jogger scrubs."

"How long can one go without water?"

Too often we underestimate the power of a *touch*, a *smile*, a *kind word*, a *listening ear*, an *honest accomplishment*, or the *smallest act of caring*, all of which have the potential to *turn a life around.*

—Leo Buscaglia, author

WHENEVER I HEAR A PERSON SAY
someone made their heart
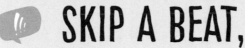 SKIP A BEAT,

all I can think is
THAT'S AN
ARRHYTHMIA
and probably should be
CHECKED OUT.

THERE'S NO ANXIETY LIKE
THE ANXIETY OF GOING BACK TO
WORK AFTER TWO WEEKS OF VACATION.

WILL I REMEMBER MY PASSWORDS?

DO I KNOW HOW TO DO MY JOB STILL?

WILL I GET THE HARDEST ASSIGNMENT?

WHAT IF MY ALARM DOESN'T GO OFF?

MURPHY'S LAW OF NURSING

#72

EVERY TIME THE HOSPITAL

BUYS NEW PATIENT BEDS,

THE FITTED SHEETS

WILL BE TOO SMALL.

NURSE FACT:

IT'S YOUR NIGHT OFF and the only clothes you know fit are SCRUBS & YOGA PANTS.

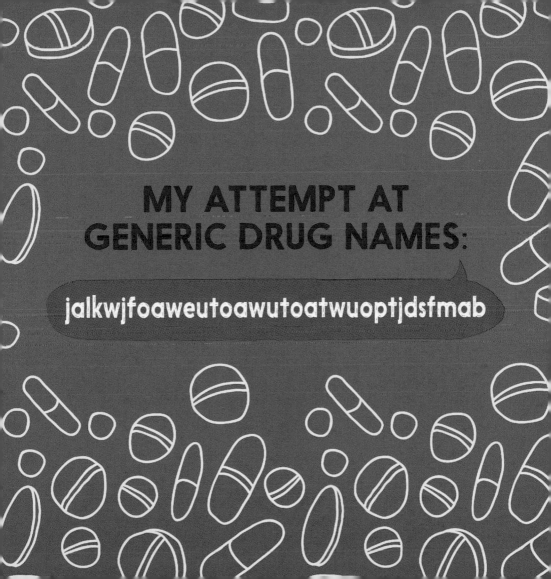

SOMETIMES

I want someone to hug me and say,

"I KNOW THIS SHIFT HAS BEEN ROUGH, BUT IT'S GOING TO BE OKAY. HERE'S SOME CHOCOLATE, COFFEE, A THERAPY DOG TO PET, AND $1.5 MILLION."

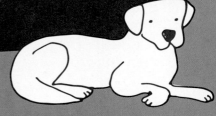

WHAT MAKES YOU THE HAPPIEST?

YOU CAN ONLY PICK ONE!

Getting a lunch break

Having your patient be adorable and thankful

Therapy dogs visiting

When your patient uses their incentive spirometer without prompting

When patients take meds via med cup instead of their hands

THERE'S NO CARDIO LIKE CHEST COMPRESSION CARDIO.

NOTHING BEATS

THE *feeling* OF

KNOWING YOU

HELPED SAVE

someone's

life.

When in doubt,
just take a deep breath.
Inhale the good stuff,
exhale the bad stuff.

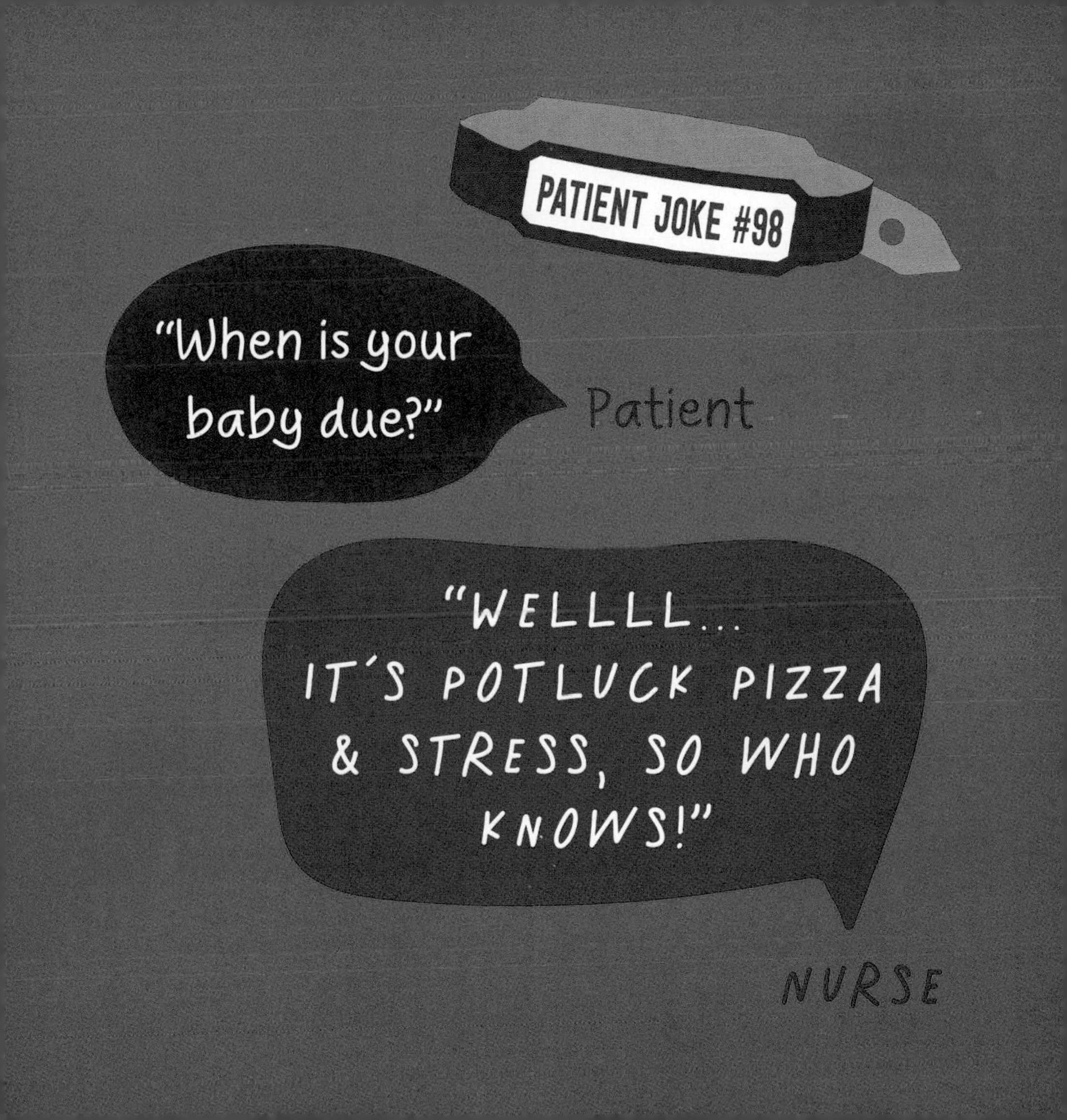
PATIENT JOKE #98
"When is your baby due?"
Patient
"WELLLL... IT'S POTLUCK PIZZA & STRESS, SO WHO KNOWS!"
NURSE

ME AS A NEW NURSE:

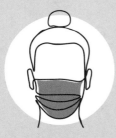

**Fifteen Minutes Early
for Shift**

New Pens in Pocket

**Pristine Scrubs in
a Fun Pattern**

**Hair in Cute
Topknot**

**Shiny Clean
Stethoscope**

ME FIVE YEARS IN:

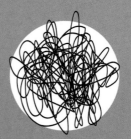

**Barely On Time
for Shift**

No Pen

**OR Scrubs from
Some Other Hospital**

**Hair Sprayed with
Dry Shampoo**

**Where's My
Stethoscope?**

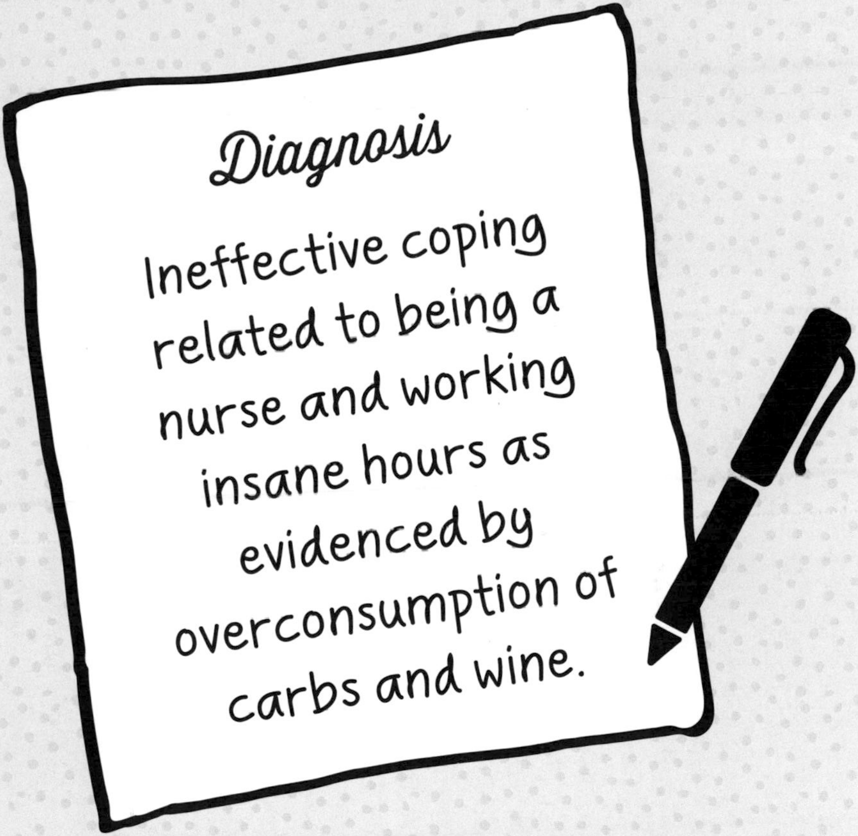
Diagnosis
Ineffective coping related to being a nurse and working insane hours as evidenced by overconsumption of carbs and wine.

Nursing:

You just have to take it one "*you've got to be kidding me*" at a time.

BE *teachable.*

BE *humble.*

BE *a team player.*

BE THE TYPE OF
NURSE YOU WANT
TO WORK WITH.

Nursing has taught me to be thankful for my health.

TINY BLESSINGS #77

When a
call light rings and
the patient says it
was an accident!

NURSING GOLD MEDAL

WHEN YOUR PATIENT SAYS THEY'RE A DIFFICULT STICK AND YOU SEE THAT FLASH OF BLOOD RETURN!

You have not lived today UNTIL YOU HAVE *done something* FOR *someone* who can never repay you.

—JOHN BUNYAN, AUTHOR AND PURITAN PREACHER

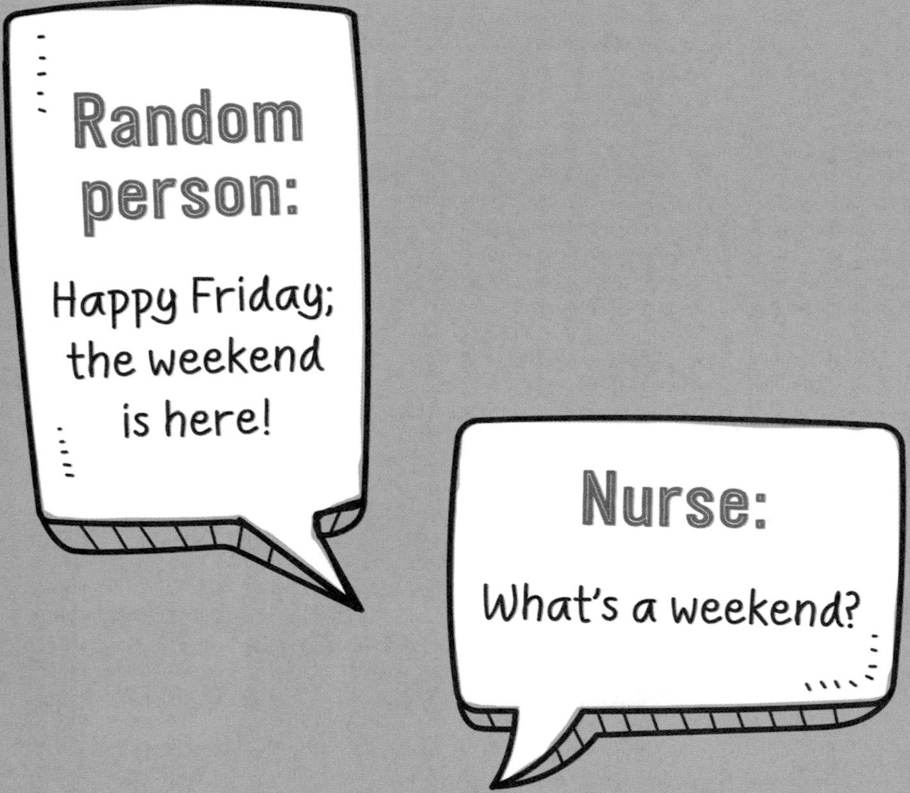
Random person:
Happy Friday; the weekend is here!
Nurse:
What's a weekend?

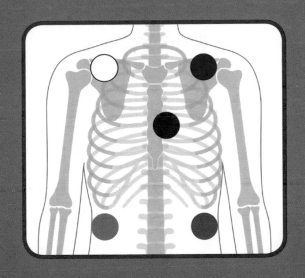

APPLYING TED HOSE IS LIKE TRYING TO **SQUEEZE** A **WATERMELON** INTO SOCKS.

BETWEEN 3–4 A.M.
ON THE NIGHT SHIFT:
WHEN EVERYTHING
IS FUNNY

Night Shift Nurses' WORST ENEMIES

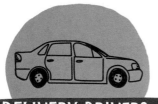

LEAF BLOWERS

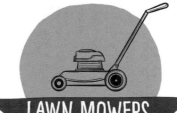

LAWN MOWERS

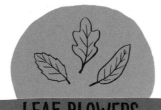

DELIVERY DRIVERS

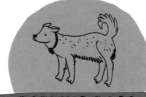

BARKING DOGS

WHEN SOMEONE
is going
through a storm,
your silent presence
IS MORE POWERFUL
than a million
empty words.

—MAHATMA GANDHI, LAWYER,
POLITICIAN, AND SOCIAL ACTIVIST

MURPHY'S LAW OF NURSING

#83

YOU PAGE THE DOC FOR
SOMETHING SUPER IMPORTANT
AND WHEN THEY CALL BACK,
YOU CAN'T REMEMBER
THE PATIENT'S NAME.

DO NO HARM, *take no* NONSENSE.

Nurses are the ♥ of healthcare.

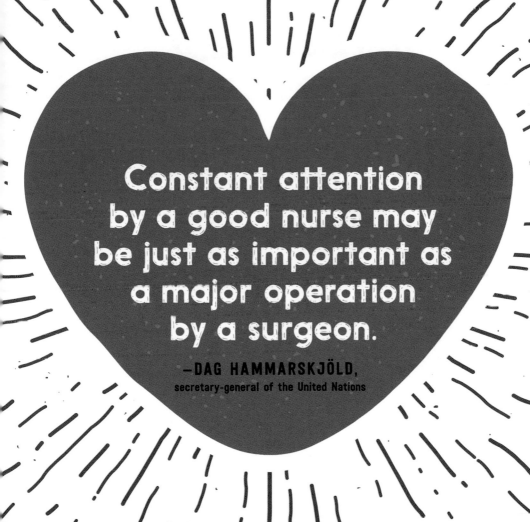

Constant attention
by a good nurse may
be just as important as
a major operation
by a surgeon.

—DAG HAMMARSKJÖLD,
secretary-general of the United Nations

You know you're a nurse if...

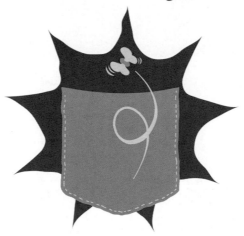

YOU'RE DIGGING IN YOUR POCKETS FOR CASH TO GET A SNACK AND ONLY COME OUT WITH CRUMPLED ALCOHOL SWABS AND A HEPARIN SHOT YOUR PATIENT REFUSED.

DOCTOR'S ORDERS THAT MAKE YOU GROAN

#88

Insert nasogastric tube on your awake patient.

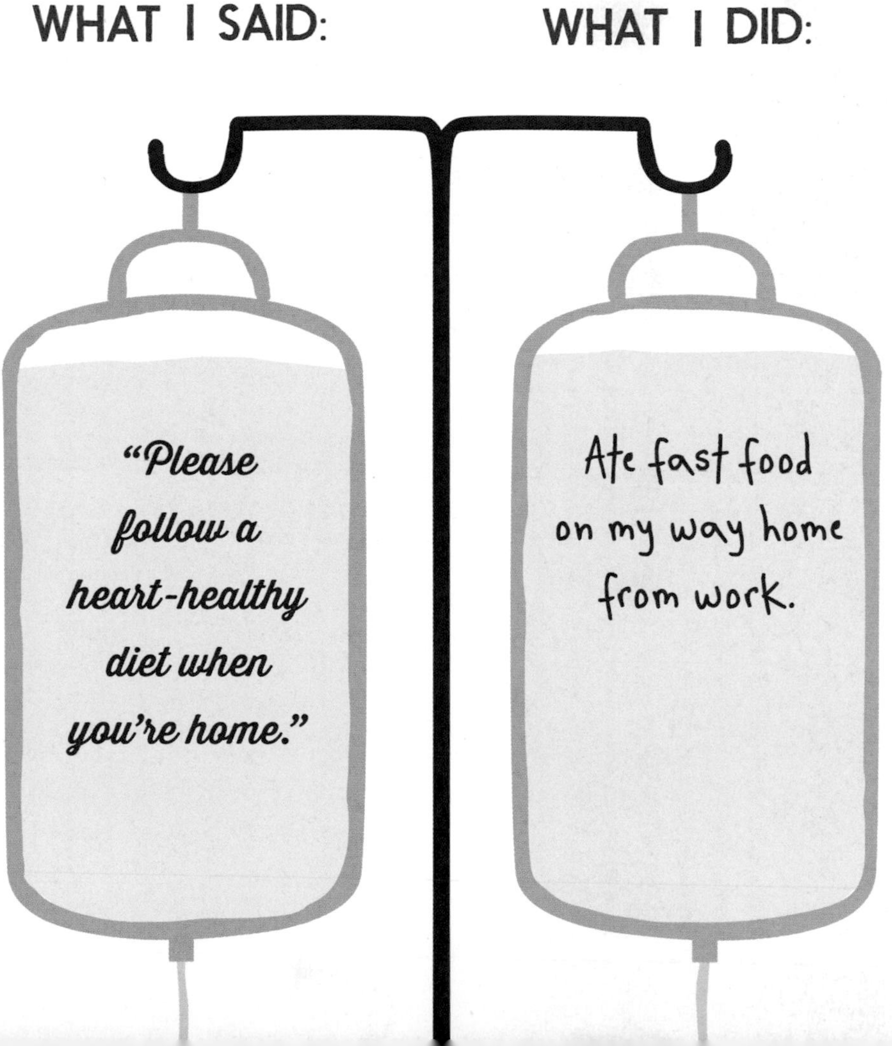
WHAT I SAID:
WHAT I DID:
"Please follow a heart-healthy diet when you're home."
Ate fast food on my way home from work.

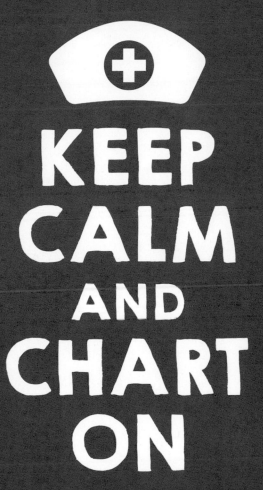

Aspire to be
THAT ONE OG NURSE
WHO KNOWS HER STUFF
AND TELLS EVERYONE
WHAT SHE THINKS
without reservation.

Nursing pet peeve #78:

Coworkers who *somehow* DON'T HEAR call lights going off.

TO KNOW *even one life* has breathed easier BECAUSE YOU HAVE LIVED. THIS *is to have* SUCCEEDED.

—Ralph Waldo Emerson, poet

A Poem about Work:

Coffee Coffee,
Meds/Walks/Alarms,
Drive home,
Wine.

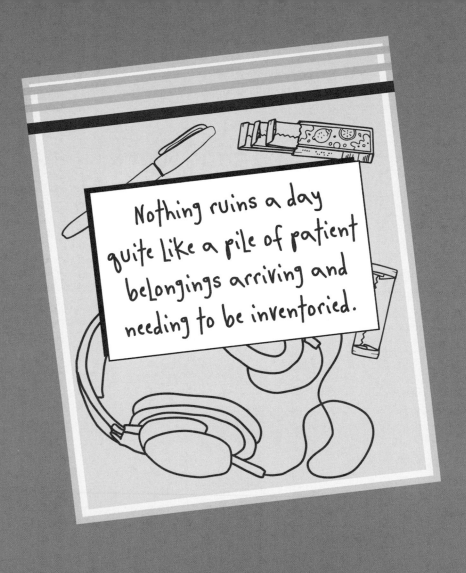

Three questions that make a nurse's eyes roll:

ARE YOU GOING TO MARRY A DOCTOR?

WHY DIDN'T YOU BECOME A DOCTOR?

WHY ARE YOU SO TIRED, YOU ONLY WORK THREE DAYS A WEEK?

You know you're getting

HANGRY

when your patient's
meal tray starts to look

appetizing.

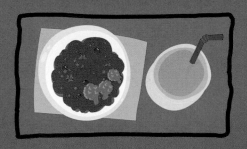

LET US NEVER CONSIDER OURSELVES FINISHED NURSES.

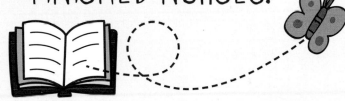

WE MUST BE LEARNING ALL OF OUR LIVES.

—Florence Nightingale,
founder of modern nursing

I'm thankful for:

coffee

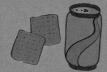

nutrition room snacks

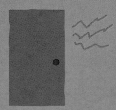

the med room where I can vent to my coworker

patients who use their call light sparingly

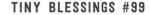

TINY BLESSINGS #99

When your patient's ID band and IV are above the covers and you can scan and hook up their IV without waking them!

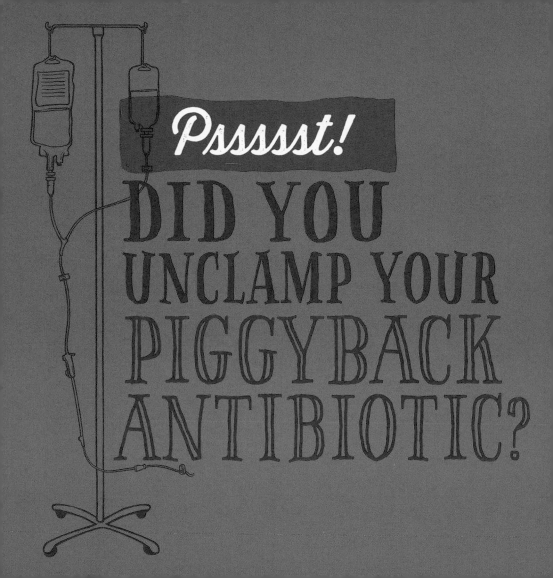

You know you're a nurse if...

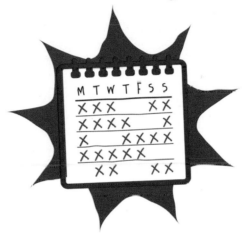

YOU'VE EXPLAINED YOUR SCHEDULE TO YOUR FAMILY A MILLION TIMES AND THEY STILL ASK YOU TO DO THINGS ON THE DAYS YOU WORK.

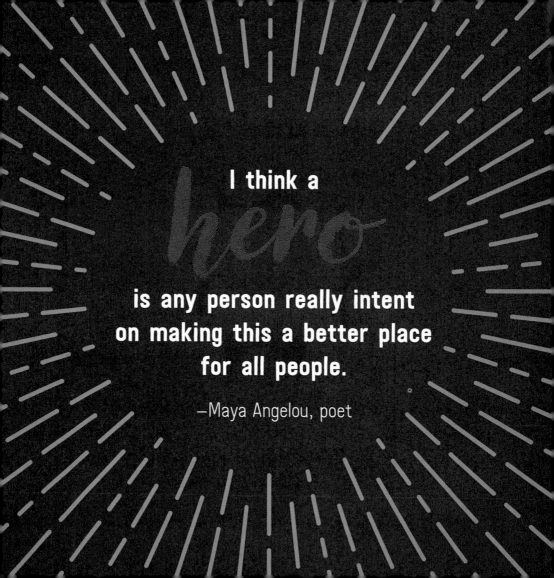

I think a

hero

is any person really intent
on making this a better place
for all people.

—Maya Angelou, poet

Lessons from Patients

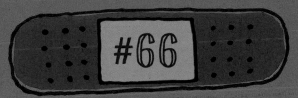

#66

IF THIS LITTLE PIGGY
STARTS LOOKING A
LITTLE STRANGE,
COME IN RIGHT AWAY!

HOW CAN ANYBODY HATE NURSES?

NOBODY HATES NURSES.

The only time you hate a nurse
is when they're giving you an enema.

—Warren Beatty, actor

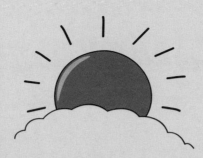

Every morning,

**make sure to take a moment
to think of all the things
you're GRATEFUL for...**

BEFORE HEADING INTO WORK
AND BEING ANNOYED
ABOUT EVERY LITTLE THING.

You know you're
a nurse if...

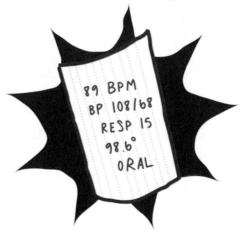

YOU USE A PAPER TOWEL TO
WRITE DOWN VITAL SIGNS.

LIVE LIFE WHEN YOU HAVE IT.

Life

is a splendid gift—

there is nothing small about it.

—FLORENCE NIGHTINGALE, FOUNDER OF MODERN NURSING

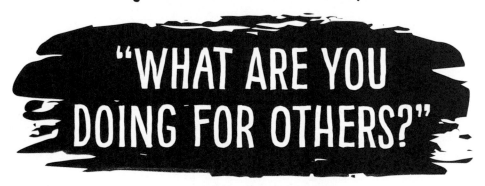

LIFE'S MOST PERSISTENT and URGENT QUESTION IS,

"WHAT ARE YOU DOING FOR OTHERS?"

—Martin Luther King Jr., minister, activist, and civil rights leader

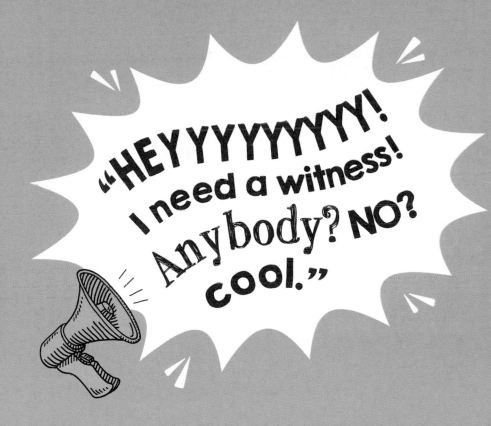

It's important to realize EACH DAY THAT A PATIENT IS PUTTING THEIR **LIFE** IN YOUR HANDS & *what a privilege that is.*

IT'S OKAY *to cry*
after a **REALLY TOUGH SHIFT.**
VULNERABILITY *AND*
SORTING THROUGH *your* FEELINGS
—— *is part of* ——
SELF-CARE.

DOCTOR'S ORDERS THAT MAKE YOU GROAN

#101

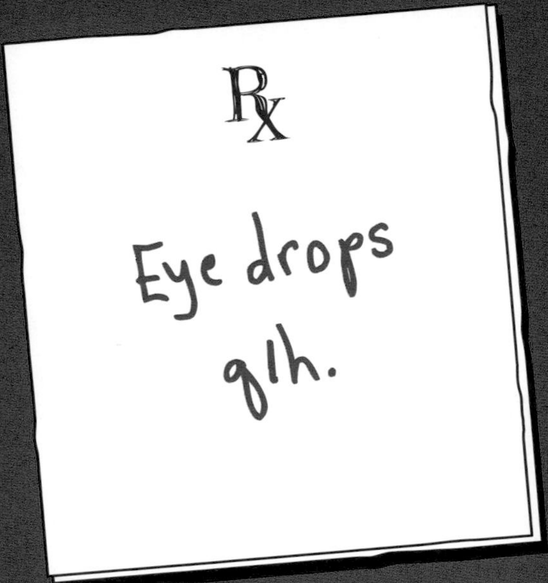

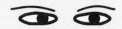

Nursing pet peeve #98:

NURSE: I have a missing antibiotic, can you send it up?

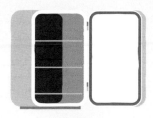

PHARMACY: Have you checked the fridge?

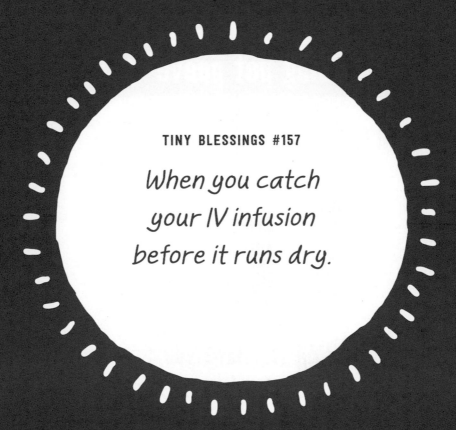

TINY BLESSINGS #157

When you catch your IV infusion before it runs dry.

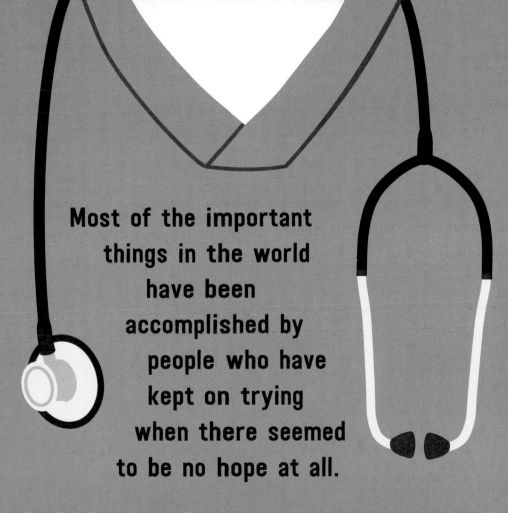

Most of the important things in the world have been accomplished by people who have kept on trying when there seemed to be no hope at all.

—DALE CARNEGIE, WRITER

YES!

I charted that I charted what I previously charted.

WAIT, HOLD ON!

I have to chart that I told you about my charting.

—AUTHOR UNKNOWN

WHAT *I love* MOST ABOUT NURSING

(SELECT ALL THAT APPLY):

- ☑ **Helping people to hopefully get back to their baseline**

- ☑ **A fast-paced learning environment**

- ☑ **Seeing the advancement of the medical world**

- ☑ **My coworkers**

- ☑ **Eating the patient snacks**

WHEN THE SHIFTS GET TOUGH,
remember why you became a nurse.